SpringerBriefs in Computer Science

Series Editors

Stan Zdonik
Peng Ning
Shashi Shekhar
Jonathan Katz
Xindong Wu
Lakhmi C. Jain
David Padua
Xuemin Shen
Borko Furht
V. S. Subrahmanian
Martial Hebert
Katsushi Ikeuchi
Bruno Siciliano

For further volumes:
http://www.springer.com/series/10028

Xiali Hei · Xiaojiang Du

Security for Wireless Implantable Medical Devices

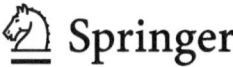 Springer

Xiali Hei
Xiaojiang Du
Department of Computer
  and Information Sciences
Temple University
Philadelphia, PA
USA

ISSN 2191-5768   ISSN 2191-5776   (electronic)
ISBN 978-1-4614-7152-3   ISBN 978-1-4614-7153-0   (eBook)
DOI 10.1007/978-1-4614-7153-0
Springer New York Heidelberg Dordrecht London

Library of Congress Control Number: 2013934023

© The Author(s) 2013
This work is subject to copyright. All rights are reserved by the Publisher, whether the whole or part of
the material is concerned, specifically the rights of translation, reprinting, reuse of illustrations,
recitation, broadcasting, reproduction on microfilms or in any other physical way, and transmission or
information storage and retrieval, electronic adaptation, computer software, or by similar or dissimilar
methodology now known or hereafter developed. Exempted from this legal reservation are brief
excerpts in connection with reviews or scholarly analysis or material supplied specifically for the
purpose of being entered and executed on a computer system, for exclusive use by the purchaser of the
work. Duplication of this publication or parts thereof is permitted only under the provisions of
the Copyright Law of the Publisher's location, in its current version, and permission for use must
always be obtained from Springer. Permissions for use may be obtained through RightsLink at the
Copyright Clearance Center. Violations are liable to prosecution under the respective Copyright Law.
The use of general descriptive names, registered names, trademarks, service marks, etc. in this
publication does not imply, even in the absence of a specific statement, that such names are exempt
from the relevant protective laws and regulations and therefore free for general use.
While the advice and information in this book are believed to be true and accurate at the date of
publication, neither the authors nor the editors nor the publisher can accept any legal responsibility for
any errors or omissions that may be made. The publisher makes no warranty, express or implied, with
respect to the material contained herein.

Printed on acid-free paper

Springer is part of Springer Science+Business Media (www.springer.com)

Preface

The objective of this book is to help readers learn more about the security and safety issues in the area of implantable medical devices (IMDs). This book takes the view that security concerns are critical in IMDs because there is the potential that a patient may be directly harmed without warning or notice. In this book, we present two plausible solutions for normal cases and emergency cases. We hope these solutions will inspire readers to propose better solutions. In addition, we review a number of current works published within the last five years. Furthermore, we discuss many future works at the end of this book, and we hope it will be helpful for researchers who are interested in this field.

In this book, we provide an overview of new security attacks, challenges, defense strategies, design issues, modeling, and performance evaluation in wireless IMDs. We mainly discuss two methods to perform access control for IMDs. One scheme is pattern-based, and the other is biometric-based.

Solutions in the book are for IMDs. This reflects both the restrictions and the specific properties of IMDs. However, we feel that it should not be difficult for researchers of other medical devices to find or construct similar solutions of their own. While studying corresponding security defenses, the readers will also learn the methodologies and tools of designing security schemes, modeling, security analysis, and performance evaluation, thus keeping pace with the fast-moving field of wireless security research.

July 2012   Xiali Hei
                                                                       Xiaojiang Du

Acknowledgments

This book could not have been written without Dr. Xiaojiang Du, who encouraged and challenged me through my academic program. He never accepted less than my best efforts. Thank you. What is written in this book are materials that I found in my papers. A special thanks to the authors mentioned in the bibliography page. I would like to acknowledge and extend my heartfelt gratitude to another advisor of mine—Dr. Shan Lin. Most especially to my family, friends, and my son, Peiheng Ni. Words alone cannot express what I owe them for their encouragement and whose patient love enabled me to complete this book. A special thanks to JieWu for comments on my editing. The book was developed from ideas originally published in the Globecom 2010, Infocom 2011, and [1]. As always it was Editor Xuemin (Sherman) Shen who provided the shelter conditions under which the work could take place: thanks to him for this and many other things.

Acknowledgments

Contents

Acronyms

CASIA   Chinese Academy of Sciences' Institute of Automation
CGMS   Continuous Glucose Monitoring System
FAR   False Accept Rate
FRR   False Reject Rate
IMD   Implantable Medical Device
RD   Resource Depletion
SVM   Support Vector Machine

Chapter 1
Overview

1.1 Wireless IMDs

Around the globe, the market for electronic IMDs is set to expand significantly. According to a study by the Freedonia Group, medical implants is a $23 billion industry in the United States in 2007, $36 billion industry in the United States in 2012, and this market is expected to increase 7.7 % annually to $52 billion in 2015, based on an increasing prevalence of chronic disorders and the introduction of new products. These products have benefited from technological advances, and growth is expected to be strong over the forecast period. Next generation devices have increased consumer's confidence in orthopedic, cardiovascular and other IMDs. Demand also benefits from the lack of alternative treatments for many chronic disorders and injuries. Furthermore, the ability of medical implants to reduce overall treatment cost for many conditions, including osteoarthritis and chronic heart failure, will continue to grow the market for these products.

In recent years, the range of available IMDs has expanded and includes cardiac pacemakers, defibrillators, cochlear implants, insulin pumps, neurostimulators and various drug delivery systems. They can be used to treat chronic ailments such as cardiac arrhythmia [2], diabetes, and Parkinson's disease. Many IMDs are enabled with wireless communication capabilities and can communicate with an external computer/reader wirelessly. Examples of IMDs include oximeters [3], defibrillators, pacemakers [4], patient monitors [5] and neurostimulators for treatment of epilepsy and other debilitating neurological disorders. Figures 1.1, 1.2, 1.3, and 1.4 show some IMDs.

1.2 Security Issues in IMDs

With the rise in use of IMDs, security becomes a critical issue, as attacks on IMDs may do harm to the patient [6]. There are a couple of attacks that an adversary may launch on IMDs. For example, pacemakers and implantable cardioverter defibrillator

X. Hei and X. Du, *Security for Wireless Implantable Medical Devices*,
SpringerBriefs in Computer Science, DOI: 10.1007/978-1-4614-7153-0_1,
© The Author(s) 2013

Fig. 1.1 Insulin pumps from [1] used with permission from Medtronic Mini-Med, Inc.

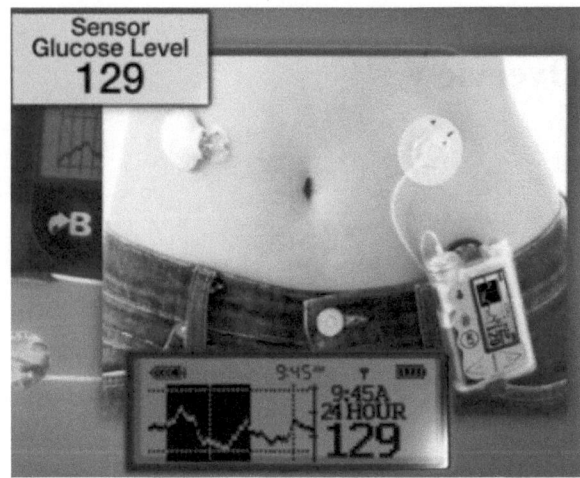

Fig. 1.2 A defibrillator. Image from [4] used with permission from Medtronic Mini-Med, Inc.

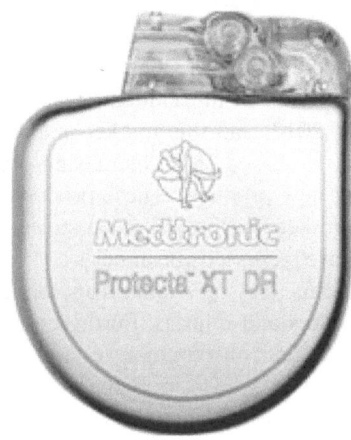

(ICDs) contain a magnetic switch that is activated by sufficiently powerful magnetic fields [7]. The current magnetic-switch-based access does not require any authentication and thus is insecure. Vulnerabilities in the communication interface of wireless programmable IMDs may allow attackers to monitor and alter the function of medical devices without even being in close proximity to the patient [8]. The consequences of an unprotected IMD have the potential to be fatal [9]. Kevin Fu et al. launched an attack against an implantable cardioverter defibrillator using a software radio to deliver a defibrillation (shock). Similarly, IBM's Jay Radcliffe presented an attack against insulin pumps in Aug. 2011. Using an easily obtainable USB device, Radcliffe [10] was able to track data transmitted from the computer and control the insulin pump's operations by intercepting wireless signals sent between the sensor device and the display device on his BG monitors; and he could cause them to

Fig. 1.3 A neurostimulator. Image from [4] used with permission from Medtronic Mini-Med, Inc.

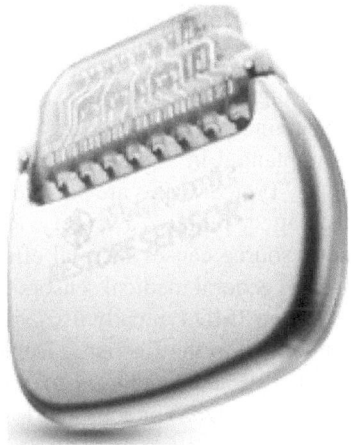

Fig. 1.4 A pacemaker. Image from [4] used with permission from Medtronic Mini-Med, Inc.

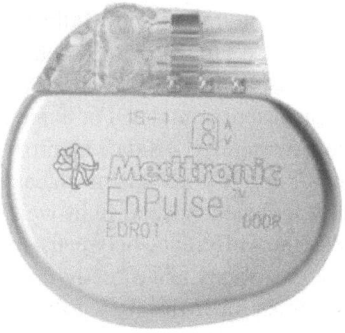

display inaccurate readings. To launch this attack, the serial number of the target device must be known beforehand. In Oct. 2011, McAfee's Barnaby Jack extended Jay's work and discovered more fatal attacks including disabling the device alarm and subsequently delivering a lethal dose without knowing the device's serial number in advance. In addition, IMDs contain sensitive patient data and information. A health insurance company may be interested in this kind of data, which could be used to increase patients' health insurance premium or even deny a patient's request.

IMD readers may be installed near the gate of a building by a malicious party, and the readers can harvest privacy information from patients' IMDs when they walk through the gate. To sum up, many attacks could be launched on IMDs, and it is critical to provide security and privacy capabilities to IMDs.

1.3 Challenges and Research Issues

Securing IMDs is a very challenging task due to their very limiting resource constraints in terms of energy supply, processing power, storage space, etc. An IMD is implanted in a patient's body and is expected to operate for several months or years. Typical IMDs are powered by a non-rechargeable battery, and replacement of the battery requires a surgery. Re-charging an IMD via an external RF electromagnetic source causes thermal effects in body tissues and thus is not recommended. Unlike general medical sensors that may use AA-type or renewable (e.g., solar) batteries, an IMD typically uses silver vanadium oxide batteries and therefore is very vulnerable to the Resource Depletion (RD) attacks [11]. The RD attacks include a number of attacks that try to consume as much energy as possible, such as Denial of Service (DoS) attacks and forced authentication attacks (discussed later). These kinds of attacks can be easily launched but are difficult to defend against. A number of literatures [12, 13, 14, 15, 16] have studied DoS attacks on wireless sensor networks. Raymond and Midkiff [14] provide a survey of DoS attacks against sensor networks. However, the security schemes designed for sensor networks cannot be directly applied to IMDs, because IMDs have much less available resources than typical sensor nodes. For example, a Mica2 mote sensor has 128 KB programmable memory and 512 K data memory [17], while an IMD may have less than 10 KB memory. Furthermore, it is much easier to replace the battery for a sensor node than for an IMD. Hence, special light-weight security schemes need to be designed for IMDs. Another difference between sensor nodes and IMDs is that an IMD is implanted in a patient's body and directly involves a human (the patient). Hence, effective security schemes for IMDs may utilize the human in their design.

During emergencies, a patient (say Bob) may be unconscious and cannot provide his credentials (such as a token or a key) to the medical personnel, nor can he show his ID or inform medical personnel about his medical information. In addition, neither device-based schemes nor family-based schemes [18] can be used if the patient has an emergency outside his home country. In this case, the safety of patients outweighs the security and privacy concerns of IMDs. A good access control scheme should satisfy security, privacy and safety requirements.

In this book, we present related works in Chap. 2, which consists of defense solutions for IMDs in normal situation as well as during emergencies. In Chap. 3, we discuss the Resource Depletion (RD) attacks and a defense scheme based on a patient's IMD access pattern. In Chap. 3, we present a light-weight biometrics based secure access control scheme for IMDs during emergencies. The conclusion and our future directions are given in Chap. 5.

Chapter 2
Related Work

2.1 Introduction

In the past several years, many research groups have dedicated themselves to security issues of IMDs. For example, Kevin Fu's group at University of Massachusetts Amherst and Fei Hu's group at University of Alabama have been working in this field for several years. There is a new conference called HealthSec Workshop that is held in conjunction with the USENIX Security Symposium. This field has attracted more and more attentions from various people, including recognitions by computer security specialists, patients, medical personnel, medical device manufactures and government regulatory agencies such as the Food and Drug Administration (FDA).

2.2 Related Work on IMD Security

There are a lot of solutions proposed to address the security issues on IMDs during normal (non-emergency) situations. Some literature propose the use of an additional external device, such as an access token [19] or a physical communications cloaking device [20]. However, these external devices may be stolen, lost, or misplaced by the patient. In addition, these devices can disclose the patient's status. Certificate-based approaches [21] require the IMD reader to be able to access the Internet, and in addition a global authority is needed to maintain certificates. The certificate-based approaches have two drawbacks: First, a reader may not always have online access. Second, it is costly to maintain a global certification authority. In [16], the authors propose allowing IMDs to emit an alert signal (sound, vibrations, etc.) when it is engaging an interaction. However, this approach may not work in noisy environments or area with barriers, and may consume excessive battery power. Some papers (e.g., [22, 23] and [24]) propose schemes that deny long distance wireless interactions with an IMD unless the proximity of the IMD is verified. For example, the secure telemetric link solution in [22] proposes the use of a physical backdoor to verify if

X. Hei and X. Du, *Security for Wireless Implantable Medical Devices*,
SpringerBriefs in Computer Science, DOI: 10.1007/978-1-4614-7153-0_2,
© The Author(s) 2013

the reader is acceptably close to the IMD. Access control based schemes on close-range communication is very intuitive, however, it is not secure against an attacker that uses special equipments (e.g., high-gain antennas), and it cannot prevent the resource depletion attacks. The authors in [24] propose a new IMD access control scheme based on ultrasonic distance bounding. The authors of paper [25] proposes using zero power (harvested RF energy) authentication, zero power notification, and sensible security of patients to protect the IMD. Our paper [11] proposes utilizing patient's IMD access pattern and designs a novel Support Vector Machine (SVM) based scheme to address the RD attacks. With the assistance of the patient's cell phone, the scheme [11] is very effective in non-emergency cases. In addition, we [26] propose utilizing a patient's biometric information to perform authentication during emergency situations. Other literature [27] proposes a wearable device called "the shield," designed to jam any incoming signals to the medical device. It doesn't require any modification to equipment the patient already has, and it is small enough that it can be easily removed for medical procedures. The built-in alarm beeps or vibrates to alert a patient or care giver of an incoming attack. This solution does not require cryptographic mechanisms and is directly applicable to IMDs that are already implanted. Using a USB device (which is used to upload the data to the web-based Carelink system) purchased from eBay, Radcliffe [9] was able to track data transmitted from the computer and control the insulin pump's operations. He found that by intercepting wireless signals sent between the sensor device and the display device on his BG monitors, he could cause them to display inaccurate readings. However, he needs to know the serial number in advance, which can be harvested using existing technology. McAfee's Barnaby Jack could furtively deliver fatal doses to diabetic patients, even the entire reservoir of insulin-300u. With software and a special and custom-built antenna designed by Jack, he can locate and seize control of any device, i.e. instruct the insulin pump to perform all manner of commands within 300 feet, even when he doesn't know the serial number. Also he can just scan for any devices in the vicinity and they will respond with the serial number of the device. Other literature [28] discusses possible attacks on wireless insulin pumps and proposes using a traditional cryptographic approach (rolling code) combined with body-coupled communication to secure device communications. Our group focus on how to detect the malicious increment of insulin dosage, how to build the audit schemes on different IMDs from different manufacturers, and how to decrypt the special communication protocols of IMD system.

2.3 Related Work on Biometrics

Biometric recognition, or biometrics, refers to the automatic identification of a person based on his/her anatomical (e.g., fingerprint, iris) or behavioral (e.g., signature) characteristics or traits [29]. This method of identification offers several advantages over traditional methods involving ID cards (tokens) or PIN numbers (passwords) for various reasons: (i) the person to be identified is required to be physically present at the point-of-identification; (ii) identification based on biometric techniques obviates the need to remember a password or carry a token. With the increased integration of computers and Internet into our everyday lives, it is necessary to protect sensitive and personal data. Biometric techniques can potentially prevent unauthorized access to ATMs, cellular phones, laptops, and computer networks. Unlike biometric traits, PINs or passwords may be forgotten, and credentials like passports and driver's licenses may be forged, stolen, or lost. As a result, biometric systems are being deployed to enhance security and reduce financial fraud. Various biometric traits are being used for real-time recognition, the most popular being face, iris and fingerprint. However, there are biometric systems that are based on more than one biometric trait such as retinal scan, voice, signature and hand geometry together to attain higher security and to handle failure to enroll situations for some users. Such systems are called multi-modal biometric systems.

The basic idea of biometric cryptosystems [30] is either binding the cryptographic key with biometric templates (i.e., codes) or generating a key directly from the template. Therefore, biometric cryptosystems can be classified into two types: key binding and key generation.

Key binding schemes need additional credentials. Key generation schemes generate some public information to assist in verification. In fingerprint recognition, there is a term named helper data—which is public information about the biometric template, and it is used to deal with the fuzziness of biometric signals during the verification phase. The public information is supposed to reveal no important information about the biometric template while at the same time it is useful in the verification phase. The three most common biometric cryptosystem schemes are: fuzzy commitment [31], fuzzy vault [32] and fuzzy extractor [33].

Fuzzy Commitment Biometric data storage must be used as less as possible, because it is not easy to cancel or revoke them when biometric templates are compromised or stolen. Juels and Wattenberg propose a biometric system in [31]. Their method is called Fuzzy commitment because a cryptographic key is decommitted using biometric data. Here, fuzziness means that a value is sufficiently close to the original to extract the committed value. However, this scheme has some shortcomings because it is based on infeasible assumptions.

Fuzzy Vault Scheme Juels and Sudan propose Fuzzy vault schemes in [32], which can be considered as an extension of the fuzzy commitment schemes. They employ a Reed-Solomon code and evaluate the codeword using a polynomial over a set of points. One practical implementation of the fuzzy vault is in the form of a secure smart-card, as proposed in [34].

In [35], the authors show that hardening the fuzzy vault scheme with a password enhances its security and provides revocability and protection against cross-matching across different biometric systems. There are fuzzy vault implementations based on a user's face [36] and hand-written signature [37]. Moreover, two important schemes based on the key binding model are proposed in (see [33, 38]). The first scheme uses the fuzzy vault scheme to bind a secret with iris images, while the second one proposes a fuzzy extractor, according to the definitions of Dodis et al. [33].

Fuzzy vault schemes have some limitations: (1) If the same biometric data is used to construct different vaults with different polynomials and chaff points, the genuine points can be easily identified by correlating the abscissa values from the fuzzy vaults of different systems. (2) The set of chaff points is bigger than the set of genuine points and an attacker may be able to substitute some points of the chaff-point set. In this way the attacker and the original user can be identified with the same fuzzy vault. (3) The non-uniformity of biometric features makes it possible to identify the genuine set from the set of chaff points by using a statistical analysis. Chang and Li have analyzed this problem in [39].

Fuzzy Extractor Scheme A Fuzzy extractor scheme is a biometric tool whose purpose is to authenticate a user using their own biometric template as a key. It works by extracting a uniformly random string S from a biometric template B in a way that is noise-tolerant. This means that if the biometric template changes to B' but remains close, the string S can still be reproduced exactly. To help the reproduction of S, the first time the fuzzy extractor is used, i.e., in the enrollment phase, it outputs a helper string H that can be made public safely without decreasing the security of S.

The role of each variable is described in the following: S is the encryption or authentication key and H is the public data stored in the database whose function is to recover S. The user's biometric template acts as the key to recover S. The fuzzy extractor process can be considered as a pair of efficient randomized procedures: Generate (Gen) and Reproduce (Rep). The correctness of the whole procedure depends on the differences between B and B'. A basic tool needed in the development of a fuzzy extractor is a secure sketch. It allows the precise reconstruction of a noisy input. On input B a procedure outputs a sketch C. Then, given C and a value B' close to B, it is possible to recover B. The sketch is secure in the sense that it does not reveal much information about B even if C is known. Thus, it is possible to store C.

2.4 Summary

Security on wireless medical devices is a relatively new research field, which is far from being well exploited. Most of the current solutions have many limitations and cannot be widely applied. Therefore, better solutions are needed. This field has also received attentions from many academic scientists and industry specialists, and it is expected to grow in the future.

Chapter 3
The Resource Depletion Attack and Defense Scheme

3.1 Introduction

Due to the limiting resources of IMDs in terms of energy supply, processor capability, and storage space, it is challenging to design efficient access control schemes for IMDs. An IMD is implanted in the patient's body and is expected remain operational for several years. Most IMDs are powered by a non-rechargeable battery, and replacing the battery requires a surgery. Re-charging an IMD from an external RF electromagnetic source causes thermal effects in body tissue and is therefore not recommended. Unlike general medical sensors that may use AA-type or renewable (e.g., solar) batteries, an IMD typically uses silver vanadium oxide batteries, and is therefore very vulnerable to the RD attacks. The RD attacks include a number of attacks that try to consume as much of the IMD's resources as possible, similar to the Denial of Service (DoS) attacks and forced authentication attacks (discussed later). The RD attacks can be easily launched and are difficult to defend against.

Ideally, an IMD should only communicate with a small number of readers (such as those in the patient's home and the Doctor's office). Furthermore, the communication should not happen at anytime (unless it is an emergency). For most patients, access to the IMD should exhibit some sort of pattern. Based on this observation, we propose to first build a model of normal patient IMD access, which can then be used to detect malicious access attempts by using the model combined with an efficient classification algorithm. If an IMD detects a malicious access attempt; it will enter a sleep mode and conserve its energy. The above scheme avoids an energy-expensive authentication process, which means it saves energy for the IMD, therefore effectively defends against RD attacks. In this chapter, we present a novel security scheme that is based on patient IMD access patterns and utilizes Support Vector Machines (SVMs). In this scheme, we use the patient's cell phone to perform most of the computations (such as SVMs). The proposed security scheme is the first line of defense, i.e., the scheme runs before any authentication procedure. If an access attempt does not pass our scheme, no authentication will be performed. This saves significant amounts of

X. Hei and X. Du, *Security for Wireless Implantable Medical Devices*,
SpringerBriefs in Computer Science, DOI: 10.1007/978-1-4614-7153-0_3,
© The Author(s) 2013

device energy. If a reader passes our scheme, it still needs to pass the authentication, which provides additional security to IMD access. We present the details of our SVM-based security scheme in Sect. 3.3.

3.2 Attack Model

In this chapter, we consider a RD attack that can be easily be launched by an attacker. The RD attack is referred to as a forced authentication attack, and it is described below. IMDs communicate wirelessly with external readers. When an external reader attempts to connect with an IMD, the first step is to perform authentication between the IMD and the reader. If the authentication does not pass, then the IMD drops communication with the reader. However, the authentication process itself requires the IMD to perform quite a few communications and computations, which consume a considerable amount of energy. If an unauthorized reader repeatedly tries to connect with an IMD, it would cause the IMD to perform multiple authentications, consuming a lot of battery power. In addition, this kind of attack generates a mass of security logs, which is itself a RD attack on the IMD's storage capability.

The forced authentication attack can be easily launched by an attacker through the use of software radio technology, as illustrated in Fig. 3.1. Through these RD attacks, an attacker could cause direct harm to a patient by exhausting the IMD's power supply. The RD attack can reduce the effective lifetime of an IMD from several years to several weeks, rendering the IMD useless, possibly even causing harm to the patient. Hence, it is critical to design both light-weight and effective security schemes for IMDs, which can defend against the RD attacks.

3.3 The Patient-Access-Pattern-Based Defense Scheme

To defend against the RD attacks, we propose a light-weight security scheme that utilizes patient IMD access patterns and Support Vector Machines (SVMs). Note that our scheme is the first line of defense, i.e., the scheme runs before any authentication procedure. Even if our scheme fails to prevent unauthorized access, an unauthorized

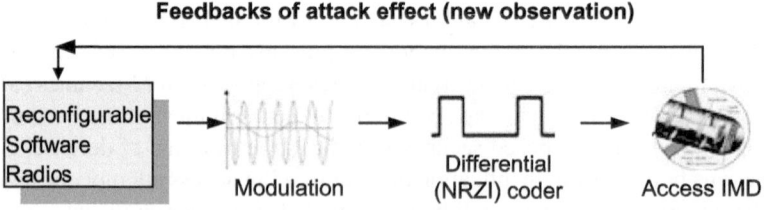

Fig. 3.1 Launching RD attacks using software radios

reader still cannot gain access to the IMD if it does not pass the authentication. We discuss the modeling of patient IMD access patterns in Sect. 3.3.1, and we present our SVM-based defense scheme in Sect. 3.3.2. Note that the focus of this chapter is on IMD access when the patient is in normal (non-emergency) conditions. In Sect. 3.3.3, we discuss the solutions for IMD access when the patient is under an emergency situation.

3.3.1 Modeling Patient IMD Access Pattern

An IMD is different from other wireless devices such as cell phones. A cell phone may have communications at any time and in many different locations. However, an IMD should only communicate with a limited number of readers (such as those in the patient's home and Doctor's office), and should not communicate with any readers at any time, with exceptions occurring only during emergency situations. For most patients, access to the IMD should exhibit a certain pattern. For example, the patient typically reads the IMD every morning and/or every evening at home. The patient's IMD typically communicates with a reader in a Doctor's office between 9 am and 5 pm. Furthermore, a particular IMD reading may have a fixed frequency, only occurring in certain locations or when certain patient conditions are satisfied. Based on the above observations, we propose an access-pattern based scheme to defend against the RD attacks. The scheme is presented below.

First, the patient's normal access pattern is obtained and utilized as training data. Second, an efficient classification algorithm is used to build a model of the patient's normal behavior. Third, the model is implemented in the patient's IMD and used to detect RD attacks in real-time.

We consider five kinds of IMD access data: reader action type, time interval of the same reader action, location, time, and day. The data is represented as a vector: $x = < a_1(x), a_2(x), a_3(x), a_4(x), a_5(x) >$, where $a_1(x)$ is the type of action that the reader wants to perform on the IMD; $a_2(x)$ is the time interval of the same action. The types of action depend on the type of IMD. For an implantable cardioverter defibrillator (ICD), the action could be one of the followings: ICD identification; obtaining patient data; obtaining cardiac data; changing patient name; setting ICD's clock; changing therapies; and inducing fibrillation. $a_3(x)$ is the location of the IMD, which has a few authorized values: e.g., home, hospital, pharmacy; $a_4(x)$ is the time of the IMD reading, e.g., 24 different values representing hours of the day; $a_5(x)$ represents the type of day, which has two values weekday, weekend. In our experimental implementations, all data is normalized to get better results.

Combining the IMD reader action type with the time interval, location and timing information can be very effective in detecting other types of attacks possible attacks other than RD attacks. For example, some actions (such as ICD identification and changing patient name) should only be performed in the Doctor's office. If these actions happen in other locations, it is probably an attack. During non-emergency conditions, most actions should have a pre-determined frequency. For example, reading the cardiac data is done once a day. If the time interval of this action is only 3 hours, it may be an attempt from an adversary at unauthorized access. The patient's cell phone may store his/her IMD access pattern, such as reading frequency and the previous time of each action.

3.3.2 The SVM-Based Security Scheme

Many modern cell phones have build-in RF reader and GPS functionality (such as e-GPS). Note that a cell phone has much more energy, computation and storage capability than an IMD. Hence, we propose shifting most computations and storage tasks to the patient's cell phone. The patient's cell phone stores related data and runs the classification algorithm. We use Fig. 3.2 to illustrate the scheme.

When contacted by a reader, the IMD first sends a short *Verification* message to the patient's cell phone. The cell phone then runs the classification algorithm, based on the reader action type, current location and time, and stored history data. The cell phone makes the following decisions with the output from the classification algorithm: (1) if the output indicates that this is a normal access, it sends a *Continue* command to the IMD, signalling to the IMD that it may continue the communication with the reader (i.e., perform the standard authentication); (2) if the cell phone

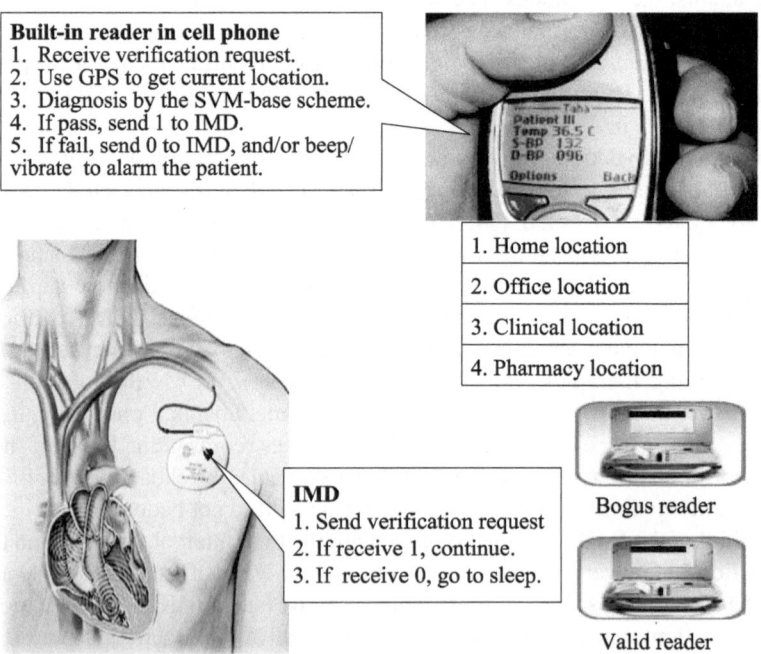

Fig. 3.2 Utilizing patient's IMD access-pattern to defend RD attacks

indicates that this is an attack, it sends a *Block* command to the IMD, and the IMD will enter a sleep mode, thereby thwarting the RD attack; (3) if the output does not have high confidence, then the cell phone may send an alarm (such as a few beeps) to the patient, and the patient may make the ultimate decision as to whether the IMD access attempt is legitimate. In (3) we utilize the human to guard against low confidence. Note that even if our scheme fails to detect an actual attack, the attacker will still need to authenticate with the device.

In our research, we designed an efficient classification scheme based on SVMs. Next, we discuss the details of using SVMs to detect RD attacks on IMDs. SVMs are efficient tools for the following task: Given some data points, and each point belongs to one of two classes, the SVM will decide which class a new data point will be classified in. Furthermore, SVMs work efficiently with small sample spaces. Hence, it is a good candidate for defending IMDs. For each SVM, there are many hyperplanes that might classify the data. One reasonable choice as the best hyperplane is the one that represents the largest separation, or margin, between the two classes. Hence, we choose the hyperplane such that the distance from it to the nearest data point on each class is maximized. A SVM can be formally represented as:

$$D = \{(x_i, y_i)|x_i \in R^p, y_i \in \{-1, 1\}\}_{i=1}^{l}, \tag{3.1}$$

where y_i is either 1 or -1, indicating the class to which the point x_i belongs. Each x_i is a p-dimensional real vector. We want to find the maximum-margin hyperplane that divides the points having $y_i = 1$ from those having $y_i = -1$. Any hyperplane can be written as the set of points x satisfying $w \bullet x - b = a, a \in [1, -1]$, where $\bullet$ denotes the dot product of two vectors. We want to choose the vectors w and b that maximize the margin. The optimization problem in primal form is formulated as follows:

$$min \left\{ \frac{\|w\|^2}{2} \right\}$$
$$subject\ to : y_i(w \bullet x_i - b) \geq 1, for\ any\ i = 1, ..., l. \tag{3.2}$$

The original optimal hyperplane algorithm—proposed by Vapnik in 1963—was a linear classifier. In 1992, Boser et al. proposed a way to create non-linear classifiers by applying the kernel trick [40] to maximum-margin hyperplanes [41]. The resulting algorithm is similar, except that every dot product is replaced by a non-linear kernel function, which was expressed by Boser et al. and Cortes et al. as the following optimization problem:

$$min \left\{ \frac{1}{2}w^T w + C \sum_{i=1}^{l} \xi_i \right\}$$
$$subject\ to : y_i(w^T \varphi(x_i) + b) \geq 1 - \xi_i, \ \xi_i \geq 0. \tag{3.3}$$

Here training vector x_i is mapped into a higher dimensional space by the function φ. Then the SVM finds a linear separating hyperplane with the maximal margin in this higher dimensional space. $C(>0)$ is the penalty parameter of the error term. In equation (3), w is also in the transformed space, and $w = \sum_i a_i y_i \varphi(x_i)$. Dot products with w for classification can again be computed by the kernel trick, i.e., $w \bullet \varphi(x) = \sum_i a_i y_i k(x_i, x_j)$. Hence, once we obtain C and γ that maximize the margin, we obtain the SVM of normal behavior. The SVM model is implemented in the patient's cell phone and is used for real-time classification of each IMD reading attempt. The kernel function $k(x_i, x_j) = \varphi(x_i)^T \varphi(x_j)$. Some common kernels include polynomial functions, radial basis functions, Gaussian radial basis functions, and hyperbolic tangent functions. In our work, we use a radial basis function as the kernel function: $k(x_i, x_j) = exp(-\gamma \|x_i - x_j\|^2)$, $\gamma > 0$.

3.3.3 IMD Access During Emergency

Note that our SVM-based scheme is designed for moderating device access under non-emergency conditions. When a patient experiences an emergency (such as a heart attack) the patient may be in any location and the emergency may happen at any time, that is, the location and/or time may not be considered to be a normal access pattern. However, emergency personnel may still need to access the patient's IMD. To resolve the conflict, we propose the following approach: When the IMD detects an emergency condition (e.g., heartbeat is above 140 beats per second), it will deactivate the SVM-based security scheme. Emergency personnel can then access the IMD without being blocked by the SVM. Another approach for providing access to IMDs in emergency situations is to use back doors engineered into the IMD. For example, a common master key may be used to access a group of IMDs. The key is secured and maintained by hospitals. Only authorized Doctors or emergency personnel have access to the master key. When an ambulance is called, the master key is obtained and carried with the IMD reader. The IMD reader will then be able to read patient's IMD.

3.4 Performance Evaluation

We conduct experiments to evaluate the performance of an SVM-based security scheme.

3.4.1 Experiment Design

We consider the case of an ICD. In our experiments, we first pre-processed the patient's access data. Recall that the patient's access data is denoted as a vector: $x = < a_1(x), a_2(x), a_3(x), a_4(x), a_5(x) >$, representing reader action type, the time interval of the same action, location, time, and day, respectively. For $a_1(x)$, we label ICD identification as 1; obtaining patient data as 2; obtaining cardiac data as 3; changing patient name as 4; setting ICD's clock as 5; changing therapies as 6; and inducing fibrillation as 7. For $a_2(x)$, we classify them to three categories. If the time interval is longer than one week, we label it as 1; if the time interval is shorter than one week but longer than one day, we label it as 2; if the time interval is shorter than one day, we label it as 3. As for $a_3(x)$, we label hospital as 1; home as 2; and pharmacy as 3. For $a_4(x)$, we label 24 different values representing the hour of the day. For $a_5(x)$, we label weekday as 0; and weekend as 1. For example, a vector $< 4, 1, 1, 9, 0 >$ means that a reader attempted to change the patient's name in the hospital at 9am during a weekday, and the last time that the patient's name was changed was more than a week ago. In our experiments, the total sample size is 3,000. We used 2,500 samples to train the SVM model, and the remaining 500 samples were used to test it. In order to obtain a better SVM model, we randomly selected the training data (2,500 samples) from the 3,000 samples, and we trained the model several times.

3.4.2 Test Results

First, we used linear classifiers for the SVM model. We ran a total of 50 tests. Table 3.1 lists the SVM parameters and the test accuracy of 10 (out of 50) tests using linear classifiers. We got best $w = (0.0938, 0.1934, -0.1340, -1.1284, 0.0460)$, $b = -3.4654$. Then, we used non-linear classifiers for the SVM model. Table 3.2 lists the SVM parameters and the test accuracy of 5 (out of 50) tests using the non-linear classifier. The highest accuracy that we got by using the optimal non-linear SVM classifier is 99.9 %, that is, only one out of 500 diagnostics was not correct. We obtained the optimal parameters $(C = 2, 048, \gamma = 2)$ for the non-linear classifier based on the data from these training tests. The optimal parameters are used to build

Table 3.1 Parameters and accuracy using linear classifier

Test	w					b	Accuracy (%)
1	0.0940,	0.1935,	−0.1339,	−1.1284,	0.0460	−3.4646	88.6
2	−0.0938,	−0.1933,	0.1340,	1.1284,	−0.0459	3.4656	90.0
3	−0.0938,	−0.1933,	0.1339,	1.1283,	−0.0459	3.4653	88.2
4	0.0944,	0.1936,	−0.1340,	−1.1285,	0.0463	−3.4637	89.2
5	0.0938,	0.1934,	−0.1340,	−1.1284,	0.0460	−3.4654	91.2
6	0.0939,	0.1934,	−0.1339,	−1.1285,	0.0457	−3.4657	89.8
7	−0.0940,	−0.1935,	0.1338,	1.1284,	−0.0459	3.4647	89.0
8	0.0943,	0.1938,	−0.1339,	−1.1286,	0.0463	−3.4635	88.8
9	0.0944,	0.1937,	−0.1341,	−1.1286,	0.0462	−3.4642	90.8
10	0.0939,	0.1936,	−0.1340,	−1.1285,	0.0461	−3.4652	88.4

Table 3.2 Parameters and accuracy using non-linear classifier

Test	C	γ	Accuracy (%)
1	2,048	2	99.9
2	512	0.5	99.4
3	8	2^{-15}	82.4
4	0.5	2	98.4
5	32	2^{-13}	84.7

Table 3.3 Summary of test accuracy of linear and non-linear classifiers using optimal parameters over 50 tests

Type	Non-linear classifier (%)	Linear classifier (%)
Lowest	93.4	88.4
Highest	99.9	91.2
Average	97.0	90.2

the optimal non-linear SVM classifier, which achieves better accuracy on most of the tests.

Table 3.3 summarizes our experimental results using linear and non-linear classifiers with optimal parameters over the 50 tests. Table 3.3 shows on average non-linear classifiers perform better than linear classifiers. Non-linear classifiers achieve an average accuracy of 97.0 %, while linear classifiers have an average accuracy of 90.2 %.

As we can see, both linear and non-linear SVM classifiers achieve high attack detection successful rate. The above experimental results show that our SVM-based security scheme is very effective in defending against RD attacks on IMD.

In the SVM-based scheme, we use the patient's cell phone to perform most of the computations. Hence, our scheme is a light-weight solution for IMDs. Since most people carry a cell phone, our scheme does not have the drawback of requiring a user to carry additional external devices. Furthermore, we utilize the human factor in our scheme. That is, when our scheme detects a possible attack, the cell phone will generate beeps or vibrate, which alarm the patient and ask the patient to verify if the access attempt is a legitimate IMD access. With the involvement of the patient, the detection rate can be further improved.

3.5 Discussions and Extensions

3.5.1 Updating SVM Parameters

If a patient moves to another location, he/she can change the home location through the cell phone. To model the access control pattern more precisely, we can update the patient access pattern according to the patient access history once every month or even once every two weeks. If a patient's cell phone becomes lost or stolen, the patient may reload the defense scheme into a new cell phone.

3.5.2 Distance-Bounding Authentication Protocol Between IMD and Cell Phone

To avoid a bogus cell phone, we use the cell phone's serial number as an authentication factor. In addition, we propose a distance-paired authentication scheme. Since the patient's cell phone is located physically near to the patient's IMD, we can allow IMDs to record the time difference from the transmission of verification request to the time a reply is received. If the time outweighs the threshold, the IMD will ignore the reply, as this cell phone may be a bogus cell phone.

3.5.3 Sleep Time

Since our goal is defending against resource depletion attacks, we can set the sleep time to 1 h or 30 min to decrease repeated authentication over an unacceptably short period of time. The sleep time is flexible and depends on the patient's access control patten.

3.5.4 How to Detect Emergency Situations

Pacemakers and implantable cardioverter defibrillators have the ability to detect heartbeat per minute of the patient. An emergency can be considered to be a heartbeat per minute larger than 120 or lower than 40. As for insulin pumps, if the blood glucose is lower than 0.5/mol, it is an emergency.

3.5.5 Jamming Attacks Between IMD and Cell Phone

Since the distance between the IMD and the cell phone is always within 1 m, jamming attacks are not easy launched. The communication between the implantable medical device and other fake cell phone will not inference the communication between the IMDs and the authorized cell phone.

Besides, we can limit the communication range of IMDs by several approaches: reducing power; placing metal objects or meshes around the IMD; and constructing special rooms or walls to block wireless signals. In addition, with the use of specialized firmware, we can limit the range of a wireless transmitter. One solution is to utilize radio-absorbing paints by painting the exterior walls of a patient's house. Anti-Wi-Fi paint contains tiny aluminum-iron oxide particles that prevent wireless signals and other radio waves from passing through. This is an effective but some kind of an extreme measure to take against snoopers and hackers.

3.5.6 *Applications*

Right now, due to the development of smart phones, IT technology specialists are about to integrate traditional medical sensors into smart phones. Thus, the patients do not need to wear so many devices with them such as blood glucose reading devices and display devices. We can imagine that the smart phones would be widely used in modern medical system in the future. Therefore, this scheme proposed by us can be used in many IMDs and real time medical system. Later on, we will work on the unified secure wireless medical framework under smart phone.

3.6 Summary

IMDs are vulnerable to the RD attacks because typical IMDs have very limited energy, computation and storage resources. In this chapter, we proposed a new security scheme that can effectively defend against the RD attacks. Our scheme utilizes the patient's IMD access patterns SVMs for real-time classification. We designed both linear and non-linear SVM classifiers, and tested their performance. Our experimental results showed that the SVM-based scheme can detect the RD attacks with very high accuracy, with an average accuracy of 90 % for linear SVMs and 97 % for non-linear SVMs. Also, our scheme can be generalized for wireless medical system with smart phone.

Chapter 4
IMD Access Control During Emergencies

4.1 Introduction

Traditional security schemes that are designed for sensor networks and other systems cannot be directly applied to IMDs, due to the severe resource constraints of IMDs, in terms of energy supply, processing capability, and storage space. For example, an IMD manufactured in 2002 (still being used today) contains as little as 8 KB of available storage [25]. Furthermore, it is not easy to replace the battery for most IMDs, as this process requires the patient to undergo a surgical procedure. Hence, it is challenging yet critical to design effective and resource-efficient security and privacy schemes for IMDs.

In our research, we design specialized light-weight security schemes for IMDs. Most IMDs are embedded in (or closely attached to) a patient's body. Based on this fact, we propose novel access control schemes for IMDs by utilizing the human factor.

A number of literatures (e.g., [19, 20, 21, 22, 23, 24, 25] and [11]) have considered access control for IMDs when the patient is in non-emergency situations. The scheme in [24] could be used for IMD access control when the patient is in an emergency situation. However, it is difficult to integrate the circuitry of the audio receiver into the circuitry of IMDs. This scheme also needs to shield the audio receiver circuit from the circuit of the IMD, which is difficult to engineer. Furthermore, when there are barriers between the patient and external monitoring equipment, its accuracy decreases dramatically.

An intuitive approach for IMD access control during emergencies is to pre-configure a backdoor key in the IMD. In an emergency, the medical personnel first need to obtain the backdoor key, and then use the key to access the IMD. However, key-based backdoor approaches have limitations. Some papers propose storing a global backdoor key on a server, and medical personnel could obtain this key via the Internet. This does not work if the unconscious patient is in another country where doctors may not have access to the server. Neither does storing the key on a hospital server. Maintaining a globally available backdoor key is costly.

X. Hei and X. Du, *Security for Wireless Implantable Medical Devices*,
SpringerBriefs in Computer Science, DOI: 10.1007/978-1-4614-7153-0_4,
© The Author(s) 2013

In summary, none of the existing IMD access control schemes work well during emergencies. In this paper, we present a novel Biometric-Based two-level Secure Access Control (BBS-AC) scheme for IMDs when the patient is in emergency situations (such as a coma).

During emergencies, a patient (say Bob) may be unconscious and therefore cannot give his credentials (such as a token and a key) to the medical personnel, nor can he show his ID to inform medical personnel about his medical information. Our main objective is to pre-configure a key based on the patient's biometrics in the IMD.

With a secure access control scheme, a doctor (who may be in another country) will be able to access Bob's IMD, obtain his identity and medical information from the IMD, and perform corresponding medical treatments. With the protection granted by the secure access control scheme, an attacker will not be able to obtain any useful information from the IMD and therefore will be incapable of causing any harm to the patient.

Biometrics is a technology used for recognition or verification of a person by using unique human physical characteristics, such as fingerprints, hand geometry, iris, and voice. Biometrics provides effective methods for identification, which can be used for access control and various security functions. It is more effective than password/PIN or smart cards due to the following traits: there is no need to memorize passwords; physical presence of the person is required; and credentials cannot be borrowed, stolen, or forgotten. Hence, it is suitable for applications in emergency situations. In our BBS-AC scheme, we utilize a patient's basic biometric information and iris image.

Our BBS-AC scheme has two levels. The 1st level uses basic biometric information, including the pattern of the patient's fingerprint, patient height, and patient eye color. The 1st level provides fast authentication that can defend against attackers who do not possess much biometric information about the patient. If an attacker passes the first level, he/she still needs to pass the 2nd level of authentication, which uses the patient's iris image. In our scheme, it is not necessary that the clinical personnel know the key or get the token in advance and it is not necessary to keep the back door keys on a global database. What the clinical institution needs is just a device to acquire the patient's iris image and basic biometric information, this solution is cheap and very easy to accomplish.

Iris recognition is one of the most precise biometric authentication methods. It is also the fastest biometric authentication method. The iris is considered to be an internal organ, which is protected by the eyelid and cornea. It is harder for an attacker to obtain a good iris image of a person, compared to fingerprints and a face image. In general, it is not easy for an attacker to get a high-quality iris image of a patient. The best way to get a detail-rich iris image is to use a near infra-red (NIR) camera. However, a NIR camera only works well when it has a distance of 50–70 cm to the person from the front. Within this range, a patient can easily detect a malicious attacker. Due to the above reasons, we choose the patient's iris image as the main biometric used in our access control scheme.

We summarize the major contributions of our work below:

1. Based on real iris data sets, we discover that there is one special bit set– Discriminative Bit Set.
2. Via experiments on real iris data sets, we demonstrate that iris recognition can be accomplished by comparing only the Discriminative Bit Set (instead of the entire iris code), which decreases the computational overhead of iris recognition by an average of 58 %.
3. We design a novel biometric-based two-level secure access control scheme for IMDs during emergencies. Our experiments on real iris data sets show that the scheme is very effective and has small overhead (suitable for IMDs). Both the FAR and FRR are close to 0.000 %.

4.2 The Biometric-Based Two-Level Access Control Scheme

Many IMDs manufactured today have incorporated certain security functions into their design. Hence, it is reasonable to assume that an IMD has basic security protections. For example, during non-emergency situations, an IMD reader still needs to pass an authentication process in order to access an IMD (e.g., reading data from the IMD). That is, all information (including patient iris data) that is pre-loaded in an IMD is protected (Fig. 4.1).

In this research, we design a novel Biometric-Based two-level Secure Access Control (BBS-AC) scheme for IMDs during emergencies. The first level employs some basic biometric information of a patient and it is discussed in Sect. 4.3. The second level access control scheme utilizes human iris images for access control and it is discussed in Sect. 4.4.

4.3 Level-One Access Control Using Basic Biometrics

4.3.1 An Overview of Biometric

A biometric system is essentially a pattern recognition system which recognizes a user by determining the authenticity of a specific anatomical or behavioral characteristic possessed by the user. To design an practical biometric system, a lot of important issues must be considered. First, a user must be enrolled in the system so that his biometric template or reference can be captured. This template is securely stored in a central database or somewhere designated to the user. The template is used for matching when identifying. A biometric system can operate either in a verification (authentication) or an identification mode on demand.

There are two ways to recognize a person: verification and identification. Verification involves confirming or denying a person's claimed identity. On the other hand, in identification, the system has to recognize a person from a list of N users in the

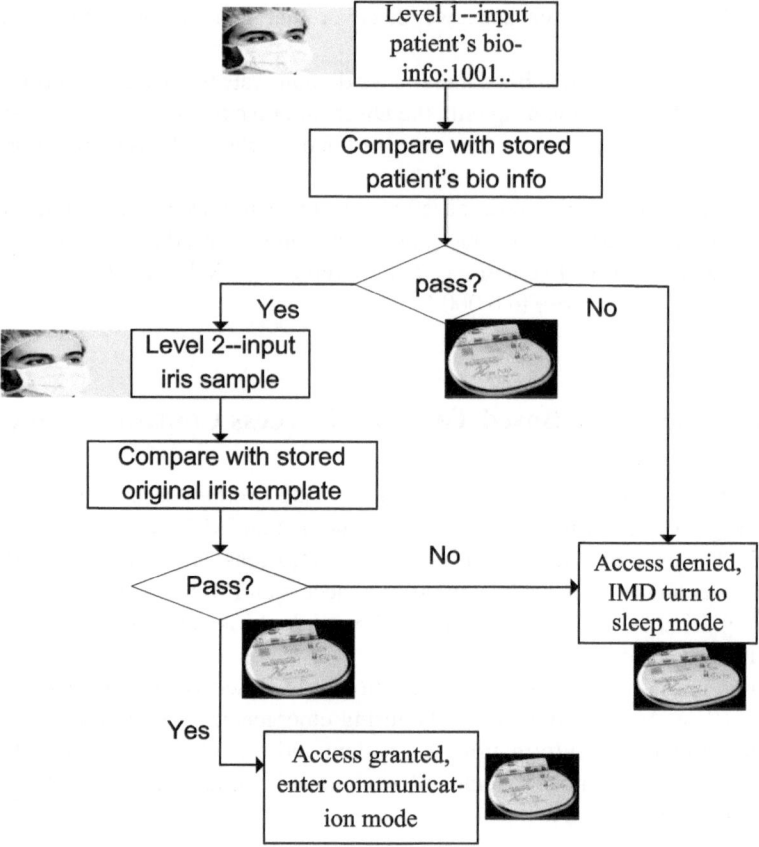

Fig. 4.1 Biometric-based two-level secure access control scheme

template database. Identification is a more challenging problem because it involves 1:N matching compared to 1:1 matching for verification.

While biometric systems, particularly automatic fingerprint identification systems (AFIS), has been widely used in forensics for criminal identification, and a large number of other civilian and government applications due to progress in algorithm and sensors. Now, biometrics is being used for physical access control, computer log-in, welfare disbursement, international border crossing and national ID cards. It can be used to verify a customer during transactions conducted via telephone and Internet (eCommerce and eBanking). In automobiles, biometrics is being adopted to replace keys for keyless entry and keyless ignition. Due to increased security threats, the International Civil Aviation Organization approved the use of e-passports.

Fig. 4.2   A front-on view of
the human eye

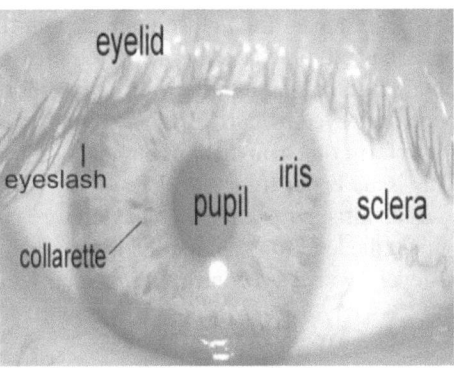

4.3.2 Suitable Biometric

A human fingerprint pattern is governed by the shape, size, and placement of volar pads [42]. Figure 4.2 shows the three fingerprint types: arch, loop, and whorl. Higher and symmetric volar pads tend to form whorls, flatter and symmetric volar pads tend to form arches, while asymmetric volar pads tend to form loops. The fingerprint types of a human does not change during the course of a human's life. Hence, we choose the fingerprint types as one of the basic biometrics in level-one. Level one uses fingerprint types of a patient's ten fingers, patient's iris color and patient's height.

4.3.3 Detailed Design

Level one uses the following three kinds of basic biometrics for access control:

- Fingerprint types of a patient's ten fingers: 0 for arch; 1 for loop; and 2 for whorl.
- Patient's iris color: 0 for dark brown; 1 for light brown; 2 for blue; and 3 for green [43].
- Patient's height.

   The three kinds of basic biometrics are relatively stable for an adult. It is not easy for an outside attacker to get all three kinds of biometric information. Hence, the level-one scheme should be able to defend against many "random" attackers. The benefits of the level-one scheme include:

- The storage required for the basic biometrics is small.
- The computation to verify the basic biometrics is light, which also means the power consumption is low.
- The verification can be done quickly (due to the above two benefits).

   Furthermore, the level-one scheme gives an authorized individual (e.g., clinical personnel) quick and easy access to an IMD during an emergency, because the clinical personnel have direct/close contact with the patient and they can easily obtain the three basic biometrics. Some extreme cases could prevent medical personnel from obtaining such biometric information. For example, the patient's fingerprints have been destroyed by burn injuries. In such extreme cases, it is probably more important to perform other medical treatments, rather than trying to access the patient's IMD. This issue is our future work.

If an attacker is able to collect all three biometrics of a patient, then he still needs to pass the level-two authentication in order to access the IMD. We discuss the details of level-two access control in the Sect. 4.4.

4.4 Level-Two Access Control Using Iris Verification

4.4.1 Challenges and Issues

Figure 4.3 is a front-on view of a human eye. Areas of the iris that are obscured by eyelids, eyelashes, or reflections from eyeglasses, or that have low contrast or a low signal-to-noise ratio lead to errors. Even through the false reject rate (FRR) and false accept rate (FAR) are very small, since the number of population is very large, the errors are sometimes recurring. Besides, how to decrease the computation of verification is very important due to the limited resources of the IMD.

4.4.1.1 Obtaining Iris Images

In case of an emergency, clinical staff can remove a patient's contact lenses and carry out strict constrains such as no eyelid and no eyelash that may shadow the iris during iris image acquisition. Thus, the error from eyelid and eyelash can be reduced dramatically.

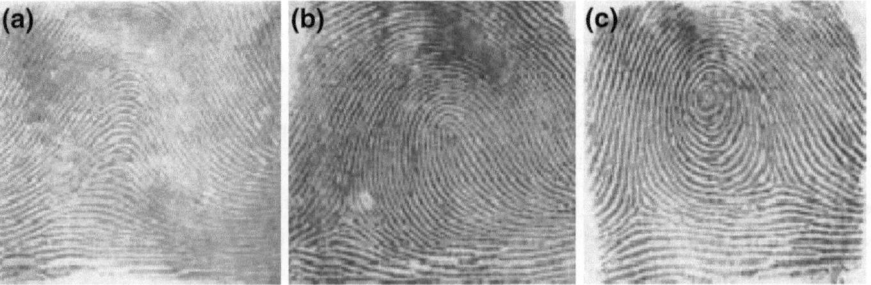

Fig. 4.3 Three fingerprint types: **a** arch **b** loop **c** whorl [19]

We use the patient's iris image as reference image during the verification, and we can acquire a sample iris image and then do the verification. For every IMD, there is only one valid iris image. Before we pre-configure the data for verification in the IMD, we select the highest quality iris image from multiple iris images (of the same patient) as a reference iris image. The IMD has severely limited computational resources, so we try to reduce the needed computation during the verification. If a color iris image is used to do verification, then we need to add a secondary step to compress the image because the color iris image is bigger than a gray iris image. In addition, NIR lighting can penetrate the iris's surface and reveal the intricate texture details that are present even in dark-colored irides. So we still use a gray iris image to do verification.

Using existing key generation methods, the false rejected rate (FRR or FNMR) is not perfect while false accepted rate (FAR or FMR) is ok. In [44], when the FAR = 1.35 %, the FRR = 11 %. This is not good for emergencies. Because safety outweighs security in case of emergency, we should not deny a genuine patient iris; so we have to reduce the FRR.

4.4.1.2 Generating Iris Codes

We store the patient's iris code θ_{ref} in the IMD before implanting the IMD into the patient's body. When the θ_{sam} is input by clinical personnel, the IMD executes the verification process. We use the schemes in [45] to get the iris code, which is 9600 bit.

Firstly, we employ an automatic segmentation algorithm (circular and linear Hough transform) to localize the iris region from the eye image. We also isolate the eyelid, eyelash and reflection areas. In addition, we can use threshold for isolating eyelashes and reflections. Next, the segmented iris region was normalized to eliminate dimensional inconsistencies between iris regions by implementing a version of Daugman's rubber sheet model. Our scheme employs Log-Gabor filters to encode iris pattern data. Finally, features of the iris were encoded by convolving the normalized iris region with 1D Log-Gabor filters and phase quantizing the output in order to produce a bit-wise biometric code. A total of 9600 bits code are calculated for the iris, and an equal number of masking bits are generated in order to mask out corrupted regions within the iris (Figs. 4.4 and 4.5).

The frequency response of a Log-Gabor filter is given below:

$$G(f) = exp(\frac{-(\log(f/f_0))^2}{2(\log(\sigma/f_0))^2}, \tag{4.1}$$

where f_0 represents the center frequency, and σ gives the bandwidth of the filter.

Fig. 4.4 The process to get
the Discriminative Bit Set

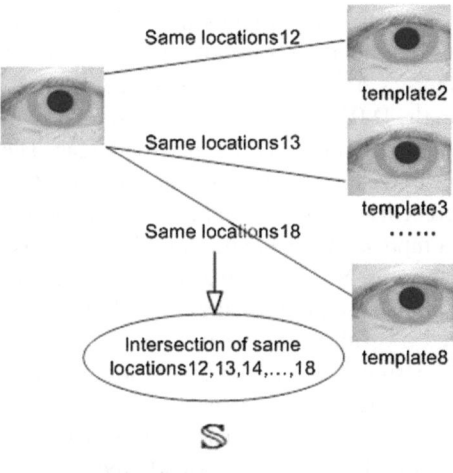

Fig. 4.5 Matching process

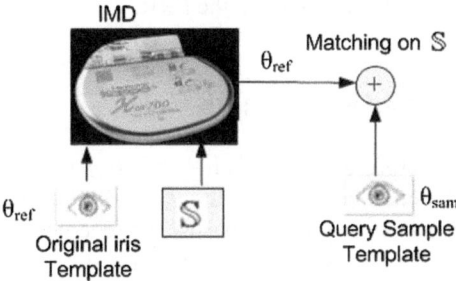

4.4.2 Discriminative Bit Set

4.4.2.1 The Discriminative Bit Set of Iris Codes

As mentioned in Sect. 4.4.1, the noise of iris codes mainly comes from areas that are obscured by eyelids and eyelashes. We focus on these two causes to reduce the noise of iris codes, which would increase the accuracy of iris verification. In our research, we wonder whether the iris codes of the same person exhibits some sort of pattern. We then try to find patterns among iris codes via experiments on several real iris data sets, including CASIA V1.0 and CASIA-IrisV3-Interval [46]. Fortunately, we are able to find one kind of special bit set among multiple iris codes of the same person. In addition, the authors of [47] first presented experiments documenting that some bits in an iris code are more consistent than others. Based on our experiments and experiments documented in [47], we realize that it is possible to perform verification by using only a small portion of the iris codes (special bit set). This greatly reduces the storage and computation requirements of iris verifications, which is significant for resource-limited IMDs. We refer to this kind special bit set as a Discriminative Bit Set.

Discriminative Bit Set—In an iris data set, each iris may have multiple images. For each iris, we choose the clearest image (denoted as image 1) as the reference image. An iris code is generated from each iris image. Recall that an iris code has a fixed length of binary bits (0 or 1). Then we compare the iris code generated from image 1 (the reference code) with iris codes generated from other images of the same iris. We record the locations of same bits (denotes as locations12 S_{12}) between the reference code and another iris code 2. Similarly, we record the same locations13 S_{13} between the reference code and iris code 3. We do this for all codes that are generated from the same iris. Suppose there are a total of k codes for the same iris. In the end, we obtain the intersection of S_{12}, S_{13}, ..., and S_{1k}. The intersection is denoted as set $\mathbb{S}$. The formal definition is given below.

Definition 4.1 $S_{ij} = \{s_{ij} \mid s_{ij}$ *is a location where iris code i and j have the same bits*$\}$

$$\mathbb{S} = S_{12} \cap S_{12} \cap ... \cap S_{1k}. \qquad (4.2)$$

If we find the invariant location set $\mathbb{S}$ among identical bits of the same iris, we can compute the hamming distance of these places between the two iris codes.

If this distance is greater than one given threshhold Th, this means these two iris codes have little probability to belong to the same iris, and they are considered to be a different identity. Otherwise, if this distance is less than the given threshhold Th, this means these two iris codes have high probability of belonging to the same iris. Through this scheme, we can decrease the computational overhead for matching schemes dramatically.

We perform experimental study on two real iris data sets (CASIA V1.0 and CASIA-IrisV3-Interval), and record the Discriminative Bit Set $\mathbb{S}$ among iris codes for each iris. Furthermore, we conduct iris-verification tests by using both the Discriminative Bit Set $\mathbb{S}$ and the entire-length iris codes. Our study shows that using only $\mathbb{S}$ for iris verifications provides similar accuracy as that of using entire-length iris codes. However, using only $\mathbb{S}$ reduces about 58 % of the computation overhead of iris verifications. We analyzed a real iris image data set CASIA V1.02, and obtained the length information of the Discriminative Bit Set $\mathbb{S}$. On average, while the ratio of $\mathbb{S}$ to the complete iris code length is 41.72 % (Table 4.1). This shows that using $\mathbb{S}$ to verify can greatly reduce storage and computation overheads.

4.4.3 Matching Scheme for Iris Codes

4.4.3.1 Uniqueness of Discriminative Bit Set

We perform several tests on real iris data sets, to ensure that the subset $\mathbb{S}$ can provide the same degree of accuracy for iris verifications as the complete iris code. The first test was to confirm the uniqueness of the set $\mathbb{S}$ for any given iris. For a given iris, there may be multiple iris codes (generated from multiple images of the same

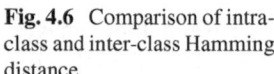

Fig. 4.6 Comparison of intra-class and inter-class Hamming distance

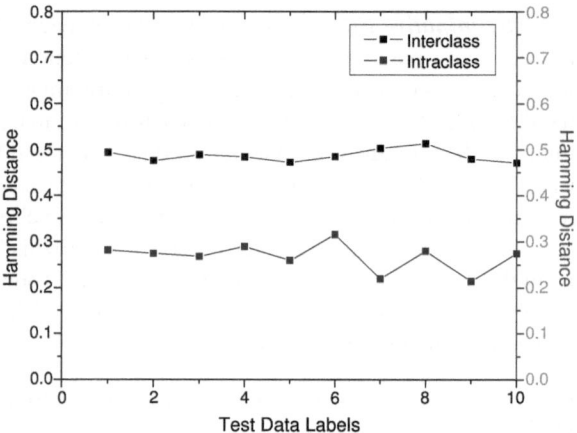

iris). However, the set $\mathbb{S}$ should be unique for any given iris/eye. This uniqueness is important since it is the foundation of accurate iris verification using the set $\mathbb{S}$. In our experiments, we confirm the uniqueness of set $\mathbb{S}$. Uniqueness was determined by comparing set $\mathbb{S}$ generated from different eyes, and examining the distribution of Hamming distance values produced. This distribution is known as the inter-class distribution [48].

Figure 4.6 shows comparisons between intra-class and inter-class Hamming distances. As we can see from Fig. 4.6: for all the tested data, the inter-class Hamming distances are always larger then 0.45; on the other hand, most intra-class Hamming distances are less than 0.3. A serial of comparisons can verify the uniqueness of set $\mathbb{S}$ in iris codes.

We use the example below to show how to obtain intra-class Hamming distances. We test V3-218-R image sets. We compare image S1218R07.jpg with S1218R01.jpg, S1218R02.jpg, S1218R03.jpg, S1218R04.jpg, S1218R05.jpg and S1218R06.jpg. Then we get the set $\mathbb{S}$. Once that is completed, we compare the set $\mathbb{S}$ of S1218R07.jpg's with the set $\mathbb{S}$ of S1218R08.jpg, S1218R09.jpg and S1218R10.jpg, obtaining 3 intra-class hamming distances. An inter-class Hamming distance is obtained by comparing the set $\mathbb{S}$ of iris codes generated from two different iris.

An essential goal of iris recognition/verification systems is to achieve a distinct separation of intra-class and inter-class Hamming distance distributions. To do this, a separation Hamming distance value (threshold) needs to be chosen. When comparing two iris codes, the threshold is used to make a decision, i.e., whether the two codes are generated from the same iris or not. If the Hamming distance between the two iris codes is less than the threshold, then the two codes are deemed to have been generated from the same iris. Otherwise, the two codes are considered to have been generated from different irises. The distance between the minimum Hamming distance value for inter-class comparisons and maximum Hamming distance value for intra-class comparisons can be used as a set threshold. Most iris matching schemes (e.g., the one in [45]) need to compare the entire iris code. In this chapter, we present a novel iris matching scheme, which only uses part of an iris code in the first step. Our scheme is based on the following observation: the iris codes of the same eye have many invariants. If the locations of invariant bits in an iris data set are relatively fixed, then we can determine the locations of discriminative bits and use the bits on these locations to perform verification. This would reduce the computation while still keeping a desired matching accuracy.

The Hamming distance is commonly used as a matching metric. In the iris verification case, a Hamming distance gives a measure of how many bits are different between two iris codes. If the hamming distance is less than the threshold, the verification is successful. Otherwise, the authentication fails. Here, we choose *fractional Hamming distances* as our matching metric.

Recall that we defined Discriminative Bit Sets $\mathbb{S}$ of an iris code. Based on the above observations and definitions, we only need to compare the set $\mathbb{S}$ of two iris codes.

There is a Hamming distance threshold (denoted as *th*) for each step. If the Hamming distance (*hd*) is greater than (or equal to) *th*, then the two iris codes are considered to have been generated from different irises, and the matching fails. If *hd* is less than *th*, then the two iris codes are considered to have been generated from the same iris. Formal definitions of the aforementioned *fractional* Hamming distances are given below.

In our work, we also perform experiments on iris codes by considering noises. Denote the Hamming distances (when considering noises) as hd. The formal definitions are given as follows:

$$
hd' = \frac{1}{m - \sum_{j \in \mathbb{S}} \theta_{refn_j}(OR)\theta_{samn_j}} \sum_{j \in \mathbb{S}} \theta_{ref_j} \bigoplus \theta_{sam_j}
(AND)\theta_{refn'_j}(AND)\theta_{samn'_j}.
\tag{4.3}
$$

Notes: m is the cardinality of set $\mathbb{S}$, θ_{ref} is the patient's reference iris code, which is stored in the IMD. θ_{sam} is the input sample iris code, which will be tested against θ_{ref}. In the above equation, j belongs to subset $\mathbb{S}$. This means that only bits of subset $\mathbb{S}$ are compared. θ_{refn} and θ_{samn} are the corresponding noise masks (the set of noise bits) for iris code θ_{ref} and θ_{sam}, respectively. And $\theta_{refn'}$ and $\theta_{samn'}$ are the complementary set of θ_{refn} and θ_{samn}, respectively. Compared with the iris matching scheme in [47], our scheme reduces the computational overhead.

4.5 Performance Evaluation

4.5.1 Experimental Data Sets

In our research, we use real iris image data sets to evaluate our scheme. The iris data sets were collected by the Chinese Academy of Sciences' Institute of Automation (CASIA). We use two data sets - CASIA V1.0 and CASIA-IrisV3-Interval. In our current experiments, we use part of the iris images from the two data sets. Specifically, we use a subset V1 (with 264 images) of the CASIA V1.0 data set, and a subset V3 (with 1,370 images) of the CASIA-IrisV3-Interval data set. The information is summarized in Table 4.2. The total number of iris images that we used is $1,634 = 264 + 1,370$, and they are generated from 198 subjects (human). For each iris, we choose the clearest iris image as the reference image, and other images of the same iris are used as training or testing data.

With these iris images, we use the algorithm in [45] to generate iris codes and the corresponding noise masks. We then perform various experiments by using the iris codes (and noise masks for some tests). The parameters chosen by us is the same as in [45], which can generate an iris code of 9,600 bits.

4.5.2 Experimental Parameters

According to [49], the optimum encoding of iris features is with one 1D Log-Gabor filter with a bandwidth given by a σ/f of 0.5. The optimal center wavelength of this filter is 18.0 pixels. An optimum code size with radial resolution of 20 pixels and angular resolution of 240 pixels was chosen for both data sets. These parameters generate a biometric code that contains 9,600 bits of information. We use these optimal parameters in our experiment.

The parameters we choose are the same as the parameters in [45], which can generate an iris code of 9,600 bits. And they are given in the following:

- Bandwidth of 1-D Log-Gabor filter: 0.5
- Center wavelength of this filter: 18.0 pixels
- Radial resolution: 20 pixels
- Angular resolution: 240 pixels

4.5.3 Experimental Results

Nextly, we present our experimental results on iris verification/ matching by using the BBS-AC scheme. In our experiments, we use FAR and FRR as metrics.

1. *False acceptance rate (FAR)*: the probability of situations where an impostor is accepted, also known in detection theory as a false alarm.
2. *False rejection rate (FRR)*: the probability of situations where a user is incorrectly rejected, also known in detection theory as a miss.

FAR and *FRR* include matching errors and biometric signal acquisition errors. Although they are convenient measures for a potential system user, they have some ambiguity because they vary if the system allows multiple attempts or has multiple templates. For this reason, matching algorithm errors are defined as those for a single

Table 4.1 The DBS percentage of a total Iris code

Data sets	L_S	L_T	L_S/L_T (%)
V1-1-2	4,415	9,600	45.99
V1-2-2	3,384	9,600	35.25
V1-3-2	5,675	9,600	59.11
V1-4-2	5,662	9,600	58.98
V1-5-2	3,281	9,600	34.18
V1-6-2	4,579	9,600	47.70
V1-9-2	2,999	9,600	31.24
V1-14-2	3,120	9,600	32.50
V1-51-2	3,358	9,600	34.98
Average	3,852	9,600	41.72

comparison of a submitted sample against an enrolled template (model). Thus, the following matching errors are defined.

False match rate (FMR): It is the expected probability that a sample is incorrectly declared to match a single randomly-selected on-self template.

False nonmatch rate (FNMR): It is the expected probability that a sample is incorrectly declared not to match a template of the same measure from the same user supplying the sample.

Therefore, false match/nonmatch rates are calculated over the number of comparisons. Furthermore, false accept/rejection rates include *failure-to-acquire rates (FTA)*, defined as the expected proportion of transactions for which the system is unable to capture a biometric signal of adequate quality. The equivalent, when a verification decision is based on a single attempt, is the following:

$FAR = (1 - FTA) * FMR,$

$FRR = (1 - FTA) * FNMR + FTA.$

Because we process strictly constrained image acquisition processes, $(FTA \approx 0)$, then

$FAR = FMR,$

$FRR = FNMR.$

In our experiment, we use *FMR* and *FNMR* to stand for *FAR*(miss detection rate) and *FRR*(false positive rate), respectively.

There is a trade-off between these metrics. For a iris verification system where a large Hamming-distance threshold (e.g., *Th*) is used, then few impostors can fool the system, but a lot of legitimate users will be rejected. On the other hand, using a small threshold works well for the legitimate users, but it is easier for an attacker to fool the system. For our IMD access control system, FRR outweighs FAR because safety outweighs security during emergencies. It would be very costly if a legitimate user (e.g., a doctor) is denied access to the IMD when a patient experiences an emergency.

Table 4.2 Eye image sets used for testing the system

Set name	CASIA V1.0	CASIA-IrisV3-Interval
Subset	V1	V3
# of Images	264	1370
# of Intra-class comparisons	308	1670
# of Inter-class comparisons	3644	52690

Tables 4.3, 4.4, 4.5 and 4.6 list our experimental results of FAR and FRR for different thresholds based on V3 data sets. As we can see from the tables, if suitable thresholds Th are selected then both FAR and FRR can be 0.000 %. In summary, our scheme is very effective.

4.6 Performance Analysis

4.6.1 Security Analysis

In the following several paragraphs, we analyze the security features of our system. Our basic design depends on two factors: an iris code and a patient's three basic pieces of biometric information. If these three basic biometrics are compromised, the iris code remains secure. The first authentication is completely independent of the iris code. It is not easy to obtain the iris code of another person. An NIR camera is needed, and it is difficult to capture a good iris image without being noticed; iris code theft is most likely be conducted using subverted equipment in falsely genuine verification settings [50]. If an attacker obtains an iris code; then our scheme rely on the first level (i.e., the three basic biometrics). The probability of the three basic pieces of biometric information being identical is:

Table 4.3 False accept and false reject rates with different threshold based on V3 data sets(no noise and 7 train images)

Th	FAR(%)	FRR(%)
0.4	1.254	0.000
0.3	0.000	0.000
0.2	0.000	6.634

Table 4.4 False accept and false reject rates with different threshold based on V3 data sets (with noise and 7 train images)

Th	FAR(%)	FRR(%)
0.04	6.323	0.000
0.03	0.000	0.000
0.02	0.000	3.346

Table 4.5 False accept and false reject rates with different threshold based on V1 data sets (no noise and 3 train images)

Th	FAR(%)	FRR(%)
0.5	46.137	0.000
0.4	0.000	0.000
0.3	0.000	0.000
0.3	0.000	6.243

Table 4.6 False accept and false reject rates with different threshold based on V1 data sets (with noise and 3 train images)

Th	FAR(%)	FRR(%)
0.25	18.639	0.000
0.20	0.000	0.000
0.10	0.000	8.728

$$pr = 1/(3^{10} \times 4 \times 255) = 6.6412e^{-8},$$
$$H = \log_2(pr) \simeq 25.85b. \tag{4.4}$$

Now let's consider the opposite case: when the three pieces of basic biometric information are stolen, but the iris code remains unknown. Correlations exist in every iris: these are partially caused by the radial structure of furrows, but some further amplitude and phase correlations are introduced by the 1D Log-gabor wavelet demodulation used to generate an iris code. The critical question is whether these correlations can be used, together with the correlations introduced by the error-correction process, to unlock the code. However, experiments on large corpora of iris codes show that a 9,600-bit iris code has 1,068 degrees of freedom [45], and that there is little systematic correlation among irises [51]. To try to set a rough lower bound on the difficulty facing an attacker who attempts to reconstruct the code, we consider the worst case and assume the attacker has a perfect knowledge of the correlations within the subject's iris code. Then the uncertainty of the iris code is only 1,068 bits. If we use $h_2 = 0.03$ (with noise and 7 training images), so the attacker is trying to find a 1,068-bit string within about $9600 * 0.03 = 288$-bit Hamming distance of the code, so let $z = 1,068$, and $w = 288$. By the sphere-packing bound [52]:

$$\mathcal{BF} \geq \frac{2^z}{\sum_{i=0}^{w} C_z^i} \simeq \frac{2^z}{C_z^w} = 2^{174}. \tag{4.5}$$

Hence, such a search will require at least 2^{174} computations. This may seem to be a small number to the crypto purist, who accustomed of thinking 512 bits as adequate. However, several factors need to be discussed. First, iris codes currently are—by a large margin—the most secure biometric available. Second, the value 2^{174} is a very conservative theoretical bound: if the attacker has little or no knowledge about how the patient's iris bits are correlated, the effort would be much larger, and with the current state of knowledge one really do not know how to correlate someone's iris bits unless we know their iris codes somehow. Third, each of the 2^{174} computations is moderately complex, and involves coding and matching. Recall that if the first attempt is not successful, then the patient's IMD will enter a sleep mode. Hence, our scheme is secure in both theory and in practice.

4.6.2 Computation Overhead

It takes *less than 1* ms to match a pair of sample and reference iris images by running Matlab on a computer with a 2 GHZ CPU and 2 GB memory. The computational overhead of our matching scheme is only about 42 % of the scheme in [45]. This kind of savings is significant for resource-limited devices, such as IMDs. Furthermore, the verification time of our scheme is short, critical during emergencies. The level-one authentication only needs to compare $(10 + 2 + 8) = 20$ bits, while the level-two authentication needs to compare about $9,600*0.42 = 4,032$ bits. From this we can see that our level-one scheme is very light-weight, and significantly reduces the computational overhead (and hence the energy consumption) of authentication.

4.6.3 Storage Requirement

The iris code that we used has a length of 9,600 bits. In addition, we need to store the bit set $\mathbb{S}$ in an IMD, and the length of $\mathbb{S}$ roughly equals 40 % of the length of an iris code. Adding the storage of the basic biometric information, we need a total of 1,680 bytes (about 1.5 K) of storage space in an IMD. This is a reasonable storage requirement for most modern IMDs.

4.6.4 Energy Consumption

A pacemaker (with a CPU of type 230) runs at 50 MHZ [53]. Hence, $(4,032 + 20)$ comparisons only takes about 0.08 ms. The energy consumed is negligible in comparison with ordinary therapy or communication.

4.7 Summary

In this chapter, we presented a light-weight secure access control scheme for IMDs for use during emergencies. Our scheme utilizes a patient's biometric information to prevent unauthorized access to the IMD. The scheme consists of two levels: level-one employs some basic patient biometric information and is lightweight; level-two uses a patient's iris data to achieve effective authentication. In this research, we also made two contributions to the area of iris recognition: (1) Based on real iris data sets, we discovered that there is one special bit sets–Discriminative Bit Set. (2) Through experiments on real iris data sets, we demonstrated that iris recognition can be accomplished by comparing only the Discriminative Bit Set (instead of the entire iris code). This decreases the computational overhead of iris recognition by an average of 58 %. The experimental results showed that our IMD access control scheme is very effective and has small overhead (suitable for IMDs). Both the false acceptance rate (FAR) and false rejection rate (FRR) are close to 0.000 %.

Acknowledgments We would like to thank Libor Masek for his source code [54] that was used to generate iris codes from iris images. We did some modifications on Masek's source code.

Chapter 5
Conclusion and Future Directions

5.1 New Attacks

IBM's Jay Radcliffe presented an attack against insulin pumps at BlackHat conference in Aug. 2011. Using a USB device (which is used to upload data to a proprietary web based management site) purchased from eBay, Radcliffe [10] was able to track data transmitted from the computer to the insulin pump and control the pump's operations. He found that he could cause blood glucose meters to display inaccurate readings by the interception of wireless signals sent between the sensor device and the display device on his blood glucose monitors. This attack requires prior knowledge of the serial number of the device, which may be harvested using existing technologies or social engineering skills.

Besides, McAfee's Barnaby Jack was able to surreptitiously deliver fatal doses to diabetic patients, up to the entire reservoir of insulin (300u). With software and a custom-built antenna designed by Jack, he was able to locate and seize control of any device (i.e. instruct the pump to perform any command) within 300 feet, even without knowing the serial number of the insulin pump. In addition, Jack was able to scan for any insulin pumps manufactured by Medtronic in the vicinity, and these pumps would respond with the serial number of the devices [55]. Existing literature [28] analyzed the possible attacks and proposed the use of traditional cryptographic approaches (rolling code and body-coupled communication) to secure the communications link between the devices. However, the Carelink USB does not utilize body coupled communications. Hence, the method in [28] is not suitable for securing communication between the Carelink USB and insulin pumps.

5.1.1 Paradigm Real Time Insulin Pump System

Figure 5.1 shows the wireless links and electronic devices in the Medtronic Paradigm real time insulin pump system. The One touch meter and sensor obtains blood glucose

X. Hei and X. Du, *Security for Wireless Implantable Medical Devices*,
SpringerBriefs in Computer Science, DOI: 10.1007/978-1-4614-7153-0_5,
© The Author(s) 2013

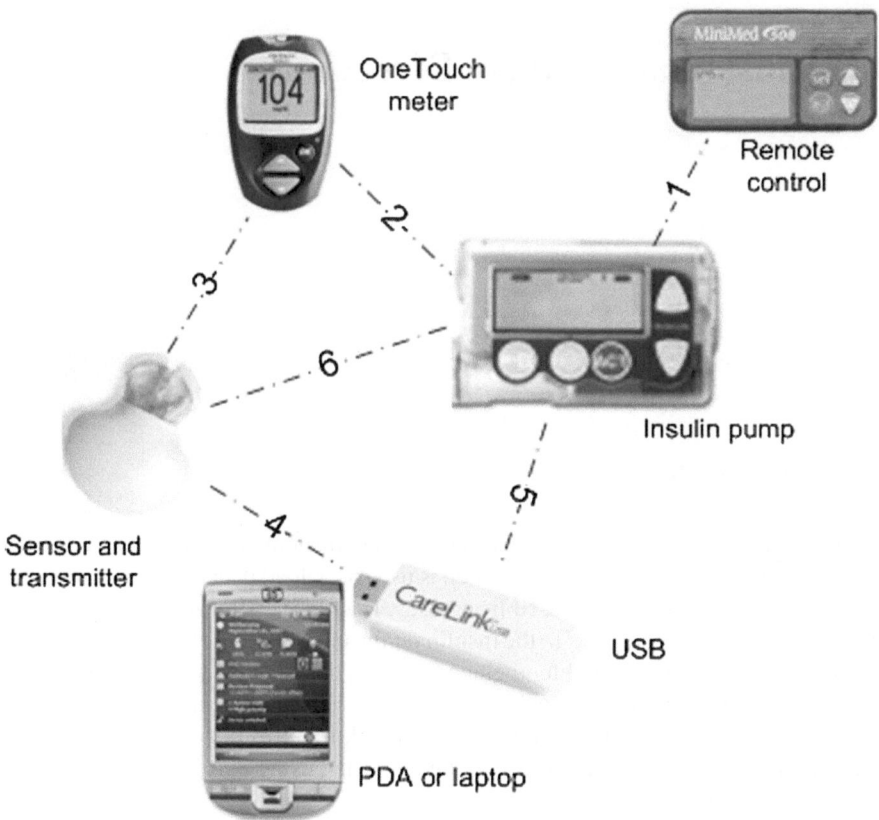

Fig. 5.1 An real time insulin pump system

readings. The insulin pump delivers insulin doses to the patient. In this system, wireless link 1 is a remote control unit sending instructions to the insulin pump. Wireless link 2 transmits blood glucose information from the blood glucose meter to the insulin pump. Wireless link 3 sends the current blood glucose reading for the sensor to the meter. Wireless link 4 transmits historical blood glucose readings to a USB device that uploads the information to a web service. Wireless link 5 allows the Carelink USB device to gather reports on blood glucose trends and patterns. Wireless link 6 sends current blood glucose levels to the pump. A laptop or PC is utilized by the Carelink USB device to upload data to a web-based management system.

5.2 Attack Analysis and Attack Model

Wireless link 1 requires a remote serial number to be provided to the pump, and the pump will vibrate/beep to confirm delivery and dosage. Since the remote control only is capable of limit operations (bolus suspend, resume), an attack on this link may not bring huge damage unless the adversary repetitively delivers the easy bolus (0.5 unit per dose) many times within a limit time that is physically encoded into the pump. Therefore, it is not easy for an attacker to perform this attack without the patient noticing and intervening.

Wireless link 2 also requires a unique serial number to be entered into the pump. The pump must be within 4 feet of a Paradigm Link meter in order to receive the blood glucose reading. One pump can accept data from a limit of 3 meters. When programming a bolus, the blood glucose measurement from the Paradigm Link meter will appear as the default blood glucose value on the ENTER blood glucose screen. If wireless link 2 is attacked, the meter and the pump would show different numbers, making the manipulation obvious.

Wireless link 5 requires a unique serial number to be entered into a computer. This link is then used to upload new settings to the pump. However, the end user software does not contain this upload capability, so an attacker would need access to the Carelink Pro software that is only legitimately available to qualified health professionals. This kind of attack would alter insulin delivery without notifying the user.

Wireless link 6 requires the serial number of the sensor to be entered into the pump. If hacked, it would report a false blood glucose level to the pump. If a level is reported that is out-of-pattern with the historical values the pump has been receiving, the pump assumes that the sensor is failing or not properly calibrated, and it therefore requires the patient manually recalibrate the sensor. This attack could harm the patient by altering insulin delivery, but this attack is not fatal without patient intervention.

In order to defend against this kind of attack, the following goals must be achieved:

- Limit the communication range of the pump.
- Securely associate the USB device, pump, and user.
- Quickly detect attacks and alert the patient.

5.3 Defending Scheme Set

5.3.1 Methods to Reduce Radio Range

We can limit the communication range of insulin pumps by several approaches: reducing power; placing metal objects or meshes around the insulin pump; and constructing special rooms or walls to block wireless signals. In addition, with the use of specialized firmware, we can limit the range of a wireless transmitter.

5.3.2 Clock Skew Scheme

Adding a timestamp to the data message, the pump can calculate the clock skew [56] by simple computation and use that to identify the other communication party. This method is very simple and efficient, but the hacker may modify his clock to falsify the timestamp or the clock skew.

5.3.3 Radio Transmitter Fingerprinting Method

Because the sensors, remote controller, meter and insulin pump all have a radio transmitter, we can use some radio transmitter fingerprinting methods (such as MoTron TxID-1 [57]) to identify the sender. However, the kind of approach may require users to add specialized and expensive devices to the insulin pump system.

5.3.4 Closed-Loop Method

To prevent wrong data being transmitted to an insulin pump, we can choose a suitable metric and add a sensor to double check the blood glucose or insulin level and send it to a Continuous Glucose Monitors System (CGMS). We can then check whether the data is valid or not.

5.3.5 Uploading Behavior Pattern

Each patient may have his own pattern as when data is uploaded. A typical insulin pump can save 3 months of logging information. The Carelink system can save all logs. From the logs, we can get the patient's uploading behavior pattern such as when he/she uploads data. For the patient, it is easy to adjust settings through the insulin pump, so he may seldom adjust the settings through Carelink USB. If we monitor the setting adjustments through Carelink USB, then we can easily detect the potential attacks.

5.3.6 Monitoring Command Setting Changes

Through reverse engineering of the java applet that the Carelink USB reader used for communications, we can get the command codes of changing settings. These commands are as listed below:

1 SETTINGINDEX_TEMP_BASAL_TYPE = 14;
2 SETTINGINDEX_TEMP_BASAL_PERCENT = 15;
3 SETTINGINDEX_PARADIGMLINK = 16;
4 SETTINGINDEX_INSULIN_ACTION_TYPE = 17;

5 CMD_TEMP_BASAL_RATE = 76 (Set Temp Basal Rate (bolus detection only);
6 MAX_TEMP_BASAL_PERCENT = 200;
7 STROKES_PER_BOLUS_UNIT = 10;
8 STROKES_PER_BASAL_UNIT = 40;
9 PUMP_NORMAL_STATE = 3;

If we log every command of type 76, 200, 14, 15, and 17, then we can monitor the setting adjustments on wireless link 5 to find out whether it is an intentional or wrong increment of basal rate and bolus dose.

5.4 Summary

As more and more patients use IMDs, it is critical to secure the wireless communication links between IMDs and remote programmers/readers. Because attacks targeting against IMDs may threaten a patient's health or even life, security schemes for IMDs should be carefully designed. In this book, we discussed state of the art in the field of security and privacy of IMDs. We hope this book will lead to more active research in this area.

References

1. [Online]. http://www.hanselman.com/blog/HackersCanKillDiabeticsWithInsulinPumpsFrom AHalfMileAwayUmNoFactsVsJournalisticFearMongering.aspx
2. J.G. Webster (ed.), *Design of Cardiac Pacemakers* (IEEE Press, Piscataway, 1995)
3. Avant 4000 bluetooth wireless oximetry: increased safety and accuracy when administering the six-minute walk test, Nonin Medical, Inc., Technical Report, 2008
4. www.medtronic.com/your-health/bradycardia/device/
5. http://www.bodymedia.com/
6. W.H. Maisel, Safety issues involving medical devices. J. Am. Med. Assoc. **294**, 955–958 (2005)
7. Implantable pacemaker and defibrillator information: magnets. Medtronic, Inc. www.medtronic.com/rhythms/downloads/3215ENp7magnetsonline.pdf
8. K. Fu, Inside risks: reducing risks of implantable medical devices. Commun. ACM **52**, 25–27 (2009)
9. D. Panescu, Emerging technologies: wireless communication systems for implantable medical devices. Eng. Med. Biol. Mag. **27**, 96–101 (2008)
10. J. Radcliffe. Hacking medical devices for fun and insulin: Breaking the human scada system. https://media.blackhat.com/bh-us-11/Radcliffe/BH_US_11_Radcliff_Hacking_Medical_Devices_WP.pdf
11. X. Hei, X. Du, J. Wu, F. Hu, Defending resource depletion attacks on implantable medical devices. in *Proceedings of the IEEE Globecom 2010*, 2010, pp. 1–5
12. K. Malasri, L. Wang, Securing wireless implantable devices for healthcare: ideas and challenges. IEEE Commun. **47**, 74–80 (2009)
13. A. Juels, Rfid security and privacy: a research survey. IEEE JSAC **24**, 381–394(2006)
14. D. Raymond, S. Midkiff, Denial-of-service in wireless sensor networks: attacks and defenses. IEEE Pervasive Computing **7**, 74–81 (2008)
15. D. Raymond, Effects of denial of sleep attacks on wireless sensor network mac protocols. in *Proceedins of the 7th Annual IEEE Systems, Man, and Cybernetics, Information Assurance, Workshop, 2006*, pp. 297–304
16. D. Halperin, T.S. Heydt-Benjamin, K. Fu, T. Kohno, W.H. Maisel, Security and privacy for implantable medical devices. IEEE Pervasive Comput. **7**, 30–39 (2008)
17. Mica2 mote sensor. Crossbow Technology. http://www.xbow.com
18. J. Sun, X. Zhu, C. Zhang, Y. Fang, Hcpp: Cryptography based secure ehr system for patient privacy and emergency healthcare. in *Proceedings of ICDCS'11*, pp. 373–382 (2011)
19. P. Inchingolo, S. Bergamasco, M. Bon, Medical data protection with a new generation of hardware authentication tokens. in *Proceedings of Mediterranean Conference on Medical and Biological Engineering and Computing*, (2001)

20. T. Denning, K. Fu, T. Kohno, Absence makes the heart grow fonder: new directions for implantable medical device security. in *Proceedings of the 3rd Conference on Hot Topics in Security*, pp. 1–7 (2008)
21. E. Freudenthal, R. Spring, L. Estevez, Practical techniques for limiting disclosure of rf-equipped medical devices. in *Proceedings of Engineering in Medicine and Biology, Workshop*, pp. 82–85 (2007)
22. U. P. A. 20080044014. Secure telemetric linksecure telemetric link. http://www.freshpatents.com
23. M.R. Rieback, B. Crispo, A.S. Tanenbaum, Rfid guardian: a battery-powered mobile device for rfid privacy management. in *Proceedings of 10th Australasian Conference on Information Security and Privacy*, pp. 184–194 (2005)
24. K.B. Rasmussen, C. Castelluccia, T. Heydt-Benjamin, S. Capkun, Proximity-based access control for implantable medical devices. in *Proceedings of ACM CCS*, pp. 410–419 (2009)
25. D. Halperin, T.S. Heydt-Benjamin, B. Ransford, S.S. Clark, B. Defend, W. Morgan, K. Fu, T. Kohno, W.H. Maisel, Pacemakers and implantable cardiac defibrillators: software radio attacks and zero-power defenses. in *Proceedings of the 2008 IEEE Symposium on Security and Privacy*, pp. 129–142 (2008)
26. X. Hei, X. Du, Biometric-based two-level secure access control for implantable medical devices during emergencies. in *Proceedings of IEEE INFOCOM 2011*, pp. 346–350 (2011)
27. S. Gollakota, H. Hassanieh, B. Ransford, D. Katabi, K. Fu, They can hear your heartbeats: Non-invasive security for implantable medical devices. in *Proceedings of ACM Conference SIGCOMM'11*, pp. 2–13 (2011)
28. C. Li, A. Raghunathan, N.K. Jha, Hijacking an insulin pump: security attacks and defenses for a diabetes therapy system. in *Proceedings of the 13th IEEE International Conference on e-Health Networking, Applications and Services*, pp. 150–156 (2011)
29. http://biometrics.cse.msu.edu/info.html
30. U. Uludag, S. Pankanti, S. Prabhakar, A.K. Jain, Biometric cryptosystems: issues and challenges. Proc. IEEE **92**(6), 948–960 (2004)
31. A. Juels, M. Wattenberg, A fuzzy commitment scheme. in *Proceedings of ACM CCS '99*, pp. 28–36 (1999)
32. A. Juels, M. Sudan, A fuzzy vault scheme. Des. Codes Crypt. **38**(2), 237–257 (2006)
33. Y. Dodis, R. Ostrovsky, L. Reyzin, A. Smith, Fuzzy extractors: how to generate strong keys from biometrics and other noisy data. SIAM J. Comput. **38**(1), 97–139 (2008)
34. T. Clancy, D. Lin, N. Kiyavash, Secure smartcard based fingerprint authentication. in *Proceedings of ACM SIGMM Workshop on Biometric Methods and Applications*, pp. 45–52 (2003)
35. K. Nandakumar, A. Nagar, A.K. Jain, Hardening fingerprint fuzzy vault using password. in *Proceedings of International Conference on Biometrics*, pp. 927–937 (2007)
36. Y.C. Feng, P.C. Yuen, Protecting face biometric data on smart-card with reed-solomon code. in *Proceedings of CVPR Workshop Privacy Research in Vision*, pp. 29–34 (2006)
37. M. Freire-Santos, J. Fierrez-Aguilar, J. Ortega-Garca, Cryptographic key generation using handwritting signature. in *Proceedings of Biometrics Technologies for Human Identifications III*, pp. 225–231 (2006)
38. Y.J. Lee, K. Bae, S.J. Lee, K.R. Park, J. Kim, Biometric key binding: Fuzzy vault based on iris images. in *Lecture Notes in Computer Science, 4642*, pp. 800–808 (2007)
39. E.-C. Chang, Q. Li, Hiding secret points amidst chaff. in *Proceedings of EURO-CRYPT 2006, Lecture Notes in Computer Science*, (2006)
40. B.E. Boser, I.M. Guyon, V.N. Vapnik, A training algorithm for optimal margin classifiers. in *Proceedings of the 5th Annual ACM Workshop on COLT*, pp. 144–152 (1992)
41. M. Aizerman, E. Braverman, L. Rozonoer, Theoretical foundations of the potential function method in pattern recognition learning. Autom. Remote Contl. **25**, 821–837 (1964)
42. M. Kuücken, A. Newell, Fingerprint formation. J. Theor. Biol. **235**(1), 71–83 (2005)
43. A.K. Jain, J. Feng, K. Nandakumar, Fingerprint matching. M. Comput. **2**, 36–44 (2010)
44. F. Álvarez, L.H. Encinas, L.S. Ávila, Biometric fuzzy extractor scheme for iris templates. in *Proceedings of WORLDCOMP'09, SAM'09*, pp. 563–569 (2009)

45. L. Masek, Recognition of human iris patterns for biometric identification. Ph.D. dissertation, The University of Western Australia, 2003
46. Casia-irisv3. http://www.cbsr.ia.ac.cn/IrisDatabase
47. K.P. Hollingsworth, K.W. Bowyer, P.J. Flynn, The best bits in an iris code. IEEE Trans. Pattern Anal. Mach. Intell. **31**(6), 964–973 (2009)
48. J.G. Daugman, Biometric personal identification system based on iris analysis. U.S. Patent 5 291 560, 1994
49. A. Ross, Iris recognition: the path forward. M. Comput. **43**(2), 30–35 (2010)
50. F. Hao, R. Anderson, J. Daugman, Combining crypto with biometrics effectively. IEEE Trans. Comput. **55**(9), 1081–1088 (2006)
51. J. Daugman, The importance of being random: statistical principles of iris recognition. Pattern Recogn. **36**(2), 279–291 (2003)
52. F.J. MacWilliams, N.J.A. Sloane, in *The Theory of Error-correcting Codes*. (North Holland, Amsterdam, 1991)
53. http://www.patentgenius.com/patent/5674259.html
54. L. Masek, P. Kovesi, Matlab source code for a biometric identification system based on iris patterns. The School of Computer Science and Software Engineering of The University of Western Australia, Technical Report, 2003
55. http://www.theregister.co.uk/2011/10/27/fatal_insulin_pump_attack
56. T. Kohno, A. Broido, K. Claffy, Remote physical device fingerprinting. IEEE Trans. Dependable Secure Comput. **2**(2), 93–108 (2005)
57. N. Serinken, K.J. Ellis, E.L. Lavigne, An evaluation of the motron txid-1 transmitter fingerprinting system. Communications Research Centre, Technical Report, 1997